CHOOSE YOU

. . .

A 40-day guide to developing healthy habits

TELIAH GIENGER

Self-Published

Washington State

2017

Contents

Cover Illustration Copyright: 2017 by Teliah Gienger
Cover picture by Melanie Faith, writer@pa.net
Book design and production by Teliah Gienger,
teliahgienger.com
Editing by Kristi Nimmo and Kylon Gienger
Inside photography by Lachelle O'Connell with Kevo
Photography

Hi friends,

I'm so glad that you are reading this book. I hope that you enjoy it as much as I did while writing it and are able to implement some of the information into your daily life. I will consider it a win if you are able to change even a tiny aspect of your health life around, due to what I have shared.

In case you don't know who I am, let me share a bit! My name is Teliah and I live in Washington state with my husband, Kylon and our pup, Sif. I am an owner in a local hot yoga studio and fresh juice bar, Renu and NUYU. During the first year of starting these businesses, I became a certified yoga instructor and finished my bachelor's degree in Health and Wellness. I love everything about living a healthy lifestyle and sharing it with my students, and now you!

Now, I didn't always be this way. In fact, despite my mother's best efforts, I wasn't terribly healthy and I hated to work out. I didn't pay attention to what foods I ate and was well overweight. It wasn't until I went to college that this began to change. I started to eat healthier, mainly because I was at a vegetarian college. I learned what being vegan was and thought people were crazy for trying, though I would try it myself just a year and a half later. I began to work out, despite my body hurting and my brain telling me to stop.

These little choices all compounded on each other to create the mindset I have now towards health. Taking these steps were essential to my life changing and I believe that by following this book and taking the tiny steps laid out for you, you can find yourself on your way to a healthier life.

Thank you for your support and I hope that this book can be a guide as well as a support for you.

How This Book Works

Here is a little tip on how this book is meant to be read.

Every day there is a goal that corresponds with the entry. It is completely up to you, but I would encourage you to try implementing the goal for that day. That first step is essential to creating a life of healthy habits.

The next day there is a new habit to mark off in addition to the previous changes. It continues until you finish this book and then it is up to you to continue implementing these habits into your daily life after the 40 days.

This is similar to 21 days of creating a habit but we will focus on 40 days to really solidify our new lifestyle.

Please keep in mind that doing all of these things right off the bat might feel overwhelming. That is not my intention with this book. Take the top 5 habits that resonate with you at this point in your life and focus on those. Then, maybe down the road a little you may find that your focus should shift and you'll come back to this book, taking something else to work on.

Again, I am your biggest fan and I can't wait to see what changes you make.

Thanks for reading and remember to choose you every day!

Food and Nutrition

Water

Our bodies are made of water so, therefore we need to drink water. Drinking water all throughout the day gives your body what it needs to function properly, ensuring that you will be at the top of your game and avoid exhaustion. Research shows that you should drink around 1 ounce of water for every pound you weigh. So, if you weigh 140 lbs, drink 140 ounces of water, or just over 4 full Nalgene water bottles a day.

Some benefits to drinking water consistently everyday include: increased energy levels and physical output, brain function, digestive health, weight loss, kidney health.

GOAL: Drink the right amount of water your body needs today.

Weight_____ = Ounces_____

Body Weight(oz) / 32 ounces = _____bottles of water a day

Calculate how much water you need to be drinking for your body, and start drinking!

Write down how many bottles of water you drank to celebrate!

Greens

If you are like me, it's difficult to eat greens in every meal. I struggle with a long-term love affair with carbs. I love them, but I know that I need to not as much. So, I really try to add greens in with my dinner especially. I can make that work so much better for some reason. Although cooking them makes them way tastier, try to eat some raw so you get all the nutrients they have to offer. Also, if you need a boost in your green intake, do what I do and add 'greens' powder to your smoothies or maybe try them plain. I love the AmazingGrass ® Green SuperFood powder or the Wheatgrass powder mixed with orange juice in the morning.

GOAL: So, for today, I want you to focus on having some greens for every meal, no matter how big or small, fresh or sautéed. JUST EAT THEM! Leafy green vegetables keep you regular with fiber, vitamin K which has some anti-aging properties, B vitamins that keep you energetic, and keep your bones strong.

In each of the sections below, choose a green that you have in your refrigerator that you can add to your meal. Keep it simple and choose just one for each meal.

Breakfast _____

Lunch _____

Dinner _____

Balanced Proportions

Eating balanced meals is essential for losing and maintaining weight. There are a lot of different sources out there that have different proportion sizes for meals. It's important to realize that our body is fueled by carbohydrates, proteins, and fats. Getting rid of any of those is not doing your body any good, you just have to learn how to proportion for your body type and what you're trying to accomplish. With that being said, studies have shown that the best way to balance your meals is by eating about 25% fiber filled carbohydrates, 25-35% protein, and 25-35% fat. Now, don't get caught up on the word "carbohydrates," as this doesn't mean just bread and pasta. A lot of vegetables are considered carbohydrates, which is why the picture below can help you to understand how much of each you actually need.

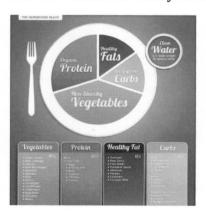

GOAL: Download the myfitnesspal app if you haven't already. Enter your information and start tracking your food intake. I do this, not to become obsessed with how much food I'm eating or not eating, but to learn how much my body actually needs to thrive. I have a tendency to put more food on my plate than I need, over-stuffing myself. Since using this app, I have become more aware of how much food I need in each category and how much I was eating before.

Sugar and Salt

Sugar and salt are the reason why food tastes so good right? Well, that may be true, but the amount of sugar and salt that the average American ingests is about 4 times the amount of salt and twice the amount of sugar that the body needs. This increased amount of salt is one of the reasons why so many Americans have high blood pressure, increased rates of heart disease, and increased risk of stroke; high sugar intake increases our risk of obesity, depression, and diabetes. It's easy to increase the amount of sugar and salt that we eat, but unfortunately it isn't as easy to cut them out. And it isn't much better to try to use substitutions because, most of the time, they contain aspartame, which has been shown to cause many other issues.

GOAL: With that being the case, for today, I'm encouraging you to not eat any added sugar or salt for an entire day and see how you feel.

Write down your mood, if you feel less or more bloated, and your overall sense of feeling.

Post that in a place you see often, so you can be reminded each time you want to eat high amounts of added sugar.

Small Meals

We are used to eating three big meals, three times a day. There is nothing wrong with this. Research shows that an issue that can arise with eating three large meals a day is the risk of having your blood sugar drop in between meals and then spike when eating your next meal. This causes a rise in insulin in the body and triggers the body to store fat quicker and easier as a coping method. Studies have shown that to prevent the spikes and valleys of insulin in the body, it's better to eat smaller meals around six times a day. This doesn't mean that your caloric intake should be any different, you are just spreading it out over the course of the day. By doing this, you prevent the dips and highs of your insulin, preventing the body from storing fat and instead burning that fat as energy.

GOAL: Below, I want you to create a meal plan for an entire day with six small meals. Keep in mind that a moderately active female should be ingesting around 1900 calories and a moderately active male around 2400 calories. This will either be more or less depending on whether you are more active or more sedentary.

Meal 1:

Meal 2:

Meal 3:

Meal 4:

Meal 5:

Meal 6:

Protein after Waking Up

Our bodies fast throughout the night as we sleep. Technically, we are still burning calories as we sleep because our body systems rely on our food's energy to keep functioning during the night. Eating a wholesome meal for breakfast is essential to managing the function of our body. By eating protein ensures we are breaking the night time fast with energy that encourages burning of fat and building of muscle. Studies have shown that most individuals ingest their main source of protein at night, which is fine, but it helps to prevent the storage of fat if protein is eaten throughout the day instead of at one meal.

GOAL: In the first 30 minutes of waking up, eat 30 grams of protein. The body just went through a huge fasting period and protein helps to sustain your body throughout the day while burning fat and building muscle.

Here are two options for early morning protein that are also easy on the stomach:

- Protein Shake with water (Already getting water intake!)
- ¼ cup of yogurt

Drink Coffee or Tea Plain

This one is pretty straight forward. We all love coffee or tea and some of us aren't ready to let that go. I get it. I love my coffee in the morning and tea in the afternoon. We are all creatures of habit so we should make sure that our habits are the best for us. A lot of Americans douse their coffee in sugar and milk. Now, I used to be one of those people that had a tiny bit of coffee in my milk and sugar. The thing is, when you drown your coffee in milk and sweetener, you're not really getting energy from the coffee. Instead, you're getting a sugar high which doesn't last for long and does crappy things to your body. Switch to plain tea or black coffee. It might be intense at first, but notice if you begin to feel different. I drink black coffee regularly, and now when I even get an Americano with soy, I feel slightly gross. Another great benefit of drinking tea and coffee plain is that they contain basically next to nothing in calories. It's a win, win!

GOAL: This morning, drink plain coffee or plain tea.

Notice how you feel and write it down on the same page as the sugar and salt page.

It's important to notice how we feel when we make changes, because if we feel good, we are more likely to continue!

Berries and Antioxidants

Berries are a power food. They are delicious, fun and can keep you healthy longer in many ways. This is due to the antioxidant power that they possess. Just by eating a few servings three or more times a week, you can harness their power for different ailments as well as losing weight. Blueberries and strawberries in particular are wonderful for keeping the mind sharp.

A few other benefits of eating berries include: Managing Diabetes, boosting heart health, weight loss and management, lowering blood pressure, urinary tract health and much more.

GOAL: Eat 1 serving of berries each day this week. It can be plain, mixed in with your morning yogurt, mixed with some almonds, blended in a smoothie, 100% fruit juice or even a homemade salad dressing like the recipe in the resource section of this book.

Trial and Error

One of the more important concepts that I love to share is the trial and error that comes with living a healthy lifestyle and maintaining a healthy diet. For six years I was a serious vegan. I felt better overall not having dairy in my diet and I never ate a ton of meat before, so it just made sense. I loved this diet for where I was at in life. I didn't have a ton of time to work out so I really had to be conscious of my diet. Fast forward to now: I'm still very much conscious of my diet, but my exercising regimen has changed drastically. I run every day and do HIIT three times a week. When I started doing this, I felt extremely weak and exhausted all the time. I knew that something needed to change because I wasn't getting all the nutrients necessary for my body. I now eat eggs on a very regular basis, though I still don't eat dairy and I'll only eat meat if I know where it came from (grass fed/organic). Even then, it's minimal. I feel 100x better on my workouts and throughout the day. All this to say, don't be afraid to change things around if they aren't working. If something works for me, it doesn't mean it will work for you and vice versa.

GOAL: Take a moment and look over your diet.

Where can something change?

What will you do to make sure that change takes place?

Don't let ego or pride get in the way. This is your life we're talking about! It took me almost a year to start eating the way I needed to, to sustain my new lifestyle and I honestly should have done it sooner.

Cheat Day

I believe that it's important to give yourself freedom through your diet and lifestyle changes, which is why I give myself a cheat day once a week. This concept has been shared over and over again through many health channels but the one that sticks out to me the most is from 4 Hour Body by Tim Ferris. It's like this: If you make a great change in your life and expect it to be executed perfectly everyday, more often than not, you exhaust yourself and the change doesn't last very long. On the other hand, if you make that same great change but allow yourself ONE day a week where you aren't as strict with that change, you are more likely to have that change last for a longer period of time. As humans, we don't like something or someone telling us that we can't have something EVER AGAIN! In fact, if you're anything like me, having someone say that makes you want it that much more. So, for the final day of our diet section, I'm telling you—no, requiring you—to create a cheat day ONCE a week. And stick to it!

GOAL: Write on your calendar your cheat day and stick to it! Easy peasy, lemon squeezy.

Physical Exercise

Move!

I'm excited to be moving into the exercise portion of this book because, although diet is extremely important, I love to exercise and I love to talk about it! When it comes to exercise, it's important to start shifting your mindset. In everything that you do today, I want you to just think, "Move". For at least 30 minutes, MOVE! If you're coming back from a severe injury or haven't worked out in a while, go for a walk; if you're normally a little more active, challenge yourself today and add an extra mile or an extra 10 min. When we begin to shift our minds to moving whenever we have a chance, our exercise and physical activity becomes a habit and like second nature.

GOAL: Move in some form for at least 30 min straight today. Go for a walk, walk up and down a hill or stairs or enjoy a workout from the back of this book!

Remember, that the thing we most often avoid is the thing we need to do the most!

Time Block

Time blocking is essential to making sure that you will get to exercise throughout the day, especially if you are a fairly busy person and your most common excuse as to why you can't workout is because, "I don't have enough time". This is where time blocking comes into play. It puts a spot on your calendar on a daily basis that is a non-negotiable. Just like we make time for social media, emails, talking on the phone, we need to make time for exercise, or else it tends to not happen. I do this for all major areas in my life, so I can ensure that it will make life easier when setting aside time for exercise. Remember that with just diet alone, you will see some results, but exercise added in will expedite the process towards living a healthier lifestyle!

GOAL: Create a reminder AND an event that occurs every day in your phone calendar right now that will ensure you get 1 hour of exercise every day!

Get Sweaty

SWEAT! Along with moving and exercising comes sweating. I love sweating and really exerting myself during my workouts. I mean, I'm a hot yoga instructor, I think I come by it naturally. But I know that some people hate the feeling of sweat on their skin and therefore won't do enough cardio to even break a sweat. Here is where I tell you to get over it, because your body needs to sweat and we all need to workout THAT hard to see the results we really want to see. Trust me when I say that once you do it, and keep doing it, you get used to sweat running down your face. If you aren't convinced just yet, here are some extra benefits to sweating daily!

1. Boosts endorphins – Feel good hormones
2. Detoxifies the skin and the body
3. Lowers kidney stone risk
4. Clears the skin – reduces acne
5. Prevents colds and other sicknesses – contains antimicrobial peptides that attack bacteria

GOAL: Workout hard enough to sweat consistently for 20 min of your hour workout each day. If you don't like to sweat yet, you will! Each day gets easier.

Injury Prevention

After being motivated to make a change in our lifestyle, it's easy to jump right into something and go full force. While that is not completely a bad thing on the emotional and mental level, sometimes it can lead to physical injury. If you are trying a new exercise or a new form of exercise, instead of jumping in full force, create a plan to work up to your desired goal. You see the importance of this with marathon runners or IronMan trainers. They don't just do the entire race on their first day of training; they set aside months to train and they have a plan for how they build up to their goal. Now, I'm just as guilty of trying to jump in too quickly without a plan, which is why I have a few apps downloaded on my phone to help. There are some great apps out there, but these are a few of my favorites:

> Couch to 5k
> Couch to 10k
> Nike+ Training Club

Remember this is important, because if you get injured, chances of accomplishing your goal go way down and you also have to wait that much longer to achieve it. Grow in your health at a steady pace and let your body catch up to your mind's goal.

GOAL: It's time to create a goal and then create your plan to reach your goal. I believe that setting goals are essential if you are wanting to see change. Dream big and don't be afraid to really challenge yourself with your goals.

Follow the goal setting worksheet guide at the end of this book for help.

Diversity is Key

Now that you have your plan and your goals, it's time to get to work. Today, we will be focusing on being diverse in our workouts. It's good to be consistent and it's extremely encouraging to be consistent in how often you are working out, but it's also essential to have diversity in your workouts. This will continue to challenge your muscles and make them stronger, quicker, and more flexible. Being diverse will also help to prevent your body from plateauing, thus preventing you from accomplishing your health goals. To help out with this, focus five days a week on cardio, three on strength training, and two on recovery/restorative practices like yoga or deep stretching. This pattern is a glimpse into my workout schedule.

GOAL: Set your workout schedule to have diverse days and make sure that on strength training days, you are focusing on different areas of the body (i.e. legs and core one day and then arms and chest/back the other day) Below is an example of what my days look like:

Monday – Cardio and Legs

Tuesday – Yoga and Core

Wednesday – Cardio and Arms

Thursday – Yoga and Core

Friday – Cardio and Full body HIIT

Saturday – Yoga and Core

Sunday – Rest Day

Shift your Mindset

I love this day! Although goals are important and they help to get the health journey started, I want to focus on the mindset of your workouts today. Having a healthy mindset is extremely important to seeing success in your exercises. Because getting healthy is not just a quick switch, but a lifestyle change, I don't want you to think about the short-term focus of 'losing weight'. I want to challenge you to think about this as a lifestyle change and the creation of habit every time you work out. This change of mindset will help to solidify the creation of this habit in your mind as something that is not something that you 'have' to do everyday but something that you want and need to do to stay healthy and keep growing your lifestyle.

GOAL: Today, along with your short-term goals, I want you to create a long-term goal. This goal will go beyond any short-term goals that you have created and really focus in on the "WHY" of your lifestyle change. Having a "WHY" behind everything you do makes you that much more inclined to accomplish the little daily goals.

Write down your "WHY" below on this page or on a separate piece of paper that you can look at often.

Rest Day

Rest days are essential in the growth, development and healing of the body and muscles. Five to six days a week, you are challenging your body and pushing it further physically than before. In order for your hard work to come to fruition, it's important to give the body a break. After stressing (working out) your muscles, in order for them to become stronger, the muscles need a chance to rebuild and grow. During your rest day, you can opt to some light yoga or stretching, but it really should be a time where you stay away from muscle building exercises. If you are looking for a way to still move your body but want to honor the rest day, go through my Yin Yoga sequence at the back of this book.

GOAL: Schedule a day, each week where you will be enjoying a total rest day from working out. Enjoy some Yin Yoga or light stretching, but avoid muscle building or endurance workouts.

My rest day is typically on Sunday. ☺

Using Bodyweight

Cardio is great for the process of beginning to lose weight. Now that your cardio should be fairly solid, in that you know you need to do it every day at least for 10 minutes, it's time to add in body weight training. We're not lifting weights—not yet—but we are going to get lean muscles by lifting our own body weight. Lifting something heavy is essential to not only the growth of your muscles but also the strength of your bones. Here are a few great benefits to bodyweight training:

-It combines cardio and weight training
-You burn fat quickly
-Continually challenging at any fitness level
-Core strength will go through the roof
-Balance and flexibility increases
-It's FREE

These are just a few reasons why bodyweight training should be at least two days of your weekly workouts. In order to get you started, download Fitness Kit App. It's only $2 and will be your most beloved app, I guarantee it. The Nike Training Club also has some great workouts that are focused on endurance training. It's free and offers great motivation.

GOAL: Schedule two to three days of bodyweight training. Download an app or work through a couple of the exercises in the back of this book. Keep up the great work!

Yoga!

I personally love this day because as most of you know, I'm a yoga instructor. Yoga is not just a time to deep stretch, although that feels really good! It's a time to do active recovery for your muscles, joints and tendons. With your new workout routine, you're throwing your muscles and your body for a loop with its new strength and that means you also have to take care of them with recovery. You can get started by going to a local yoga studio, which I highly recommend because the instructors can help with any individual challenges you may be facing. Another great resource for yoga that you can do at home for any length of time is through the website doyogawithme.com. It has very put-together videos for any kind of yoga you may be looking for.

GOAL: Do yoga for at least 30 min today and another day this week. Try to do it two-three times a week! I typically enjoy 3 days of yoga, but remember that yoga can be incorporated in basic daily routine things, like tying your shoes. Just hang out a little longer in the forward fold. ☺ You can also enjoy the sequence at the end of this book for some guidance.

Accountability Partners

Having an accountability partner is essential to creating a habit. This person is the one who will be brutally honest with you about your goals and keep you responsible to them because they want to see you succeed more than be nice to you. If you have someone in mind, that's great! Schedule three times a week to work out with them or check in with them on your progress. If you can't seem to track down a good accountability partner, feel free to reach out to me! I would love to help you with your health habit goals. You can reach me at teliahgienger.com

GOAL: Set up a schedule with an accountability partner at least 2-3 times a week. A great feature in the MyFitnessPal app is that you can share your accomplishments/workouts/meals with friends and family. So, communicate about your struggles and your achievements and keep pressing forward in your goals.

YOU ARE HALFWAY THROUGH THIS BOOK AND WELL ON YOUR WAY TO CREATING HEALTHY LIFESTYLE HABITS.

KEEP UP THE AMAZING WORK!

Mind and Emotion

Meditate

Meditation is a beneficial practice that I believe everyone should be applying in their daily lives. It does not have to be anything extra spiritual if that is not your preference, or it can be! Meditation at its core is focusing on breath, focusing on stillness, acknowledging thoughts but not letting them control us. Meditation is a great way to take a break from "input" coming into your mind. Here are just a few benefits to meditation and why it's good for your mind and body.

1. Decreases depression and anxiety
2. Increases grey matter concentration in the brain
3. Improves focus, attention, and ability to work under stress
4. Increases mental strength and resilience
5. Reduces blood pressure, the risk of heart disease, and stroke

I love meditation but I wasn't always able to sit still for longer periods of time. It took practice and building up. But since I have started, I have noticed the above benefits and much more.

GOAL: Start with five minutes and sit still in mindful meditation. Build up from there. Add a minute every day and see how long you can sit in silence with no fidgeting. Set a timer so you can be sure that you're letting your mind, as well as your physical body, rest. Another great option is the Headspace app, which will guide you through 10 minute meditations every morning.

Brain Dump/Thought Purge

Journaling is a great tool for creating excellent mental health. Brain Dumping is a term that signifies the letting go of all random or not so random thoughts onto a piece of paper so that your mind is freed up to think about what you really want to focus on, or just be clear of thought so you can meditate. We use so much of our brainpower to think throughout the day, so it's important that we are creating space to focus and think on what matters most. Plus, it's like a purge of all 'crap' or 'garbage' from days past allowing you to think presently and forward. What "Brain Dumping" looks like for me is, opening my journal, writing the date and simply starting to write down everything that is in my head. As I write down my thoughts, I allow them to pass from my brain to the sheet of paper. These thoughts can be ideas, challenges, blessings, truly anything that crosses your thoughts, write them down. Then, once you are done, close your journal and let those thoughts remain on the sheet of paper.

GOAL: Before meditating, take five minutes and do a brain dump or thought purge into your journal. Then go into your meditation session and notice any differences or clarity of mind that you may be experiencing.

Gratitude Journal

Living with a grateful mindset and heart is something that I firmly believe in. Life is so naturally polluted with negativity, sadness, and ungratefulness that it's important to counteract it in our personal lives. You are going to start a gratitude journal or an "Awesome Jar". This journal is something that I started writing in over a year ago and I continue to write in almost every morning. I believe there is always something to be grateful for, big and small, significant and insignificant. If you are wanting to go with the jar concept, have a jar set up in a place you see it every day and anytime something "awesome" happens, big or small, write it on a piece of paper with the date and put it in the jar. At the end of the year, look back on all of your awesome moments! My husband and I started this at the beginning of 2017 and love it because it requires our whole family to get involved. When we begin to focus on the grateful moments, things, and people in our lives, we begin to find more and more to be joyful, happy, and grateful about. It's simple. What you focus on is what you get. So let's focus on grateful acts!

GOAL: Today, you are going to start a gratitude journal or awesome jar. You can use a physical paper journal or you can create a note in the notes section of your phone or even use Evernote.

Whatever form you choose, every morning, think of three things/people/moments/thoughts you are grateful for and write them down. Once you do that, GREAT JOB! You just started your day with gratefulness in your mind and heart. Now, here comes the fun part. As you go through each day forward, try not to have any repeats. Try every day to think of something NEW to be grateful for.

Positive Affirmations

Just like yesterday, with creating a gratitude journal, it's important to speak positive, life-affirming statements about yourself each day. No, this isn't to puff up your chest or give you a big head, but to affirm in your mind and being that you are a good, healthy person that is changing your world for the better. These are "I am" statements as opposed to "I want to be" or "I will be". If you speak "I am," you already believe it to be true and are affirming it, whether it has completely come to fruition in your life or not.

GOAL: Today, take some time and write down ten affirmations about yourself and your life. Really try to go deep. Avoid statements like, "I am a good person." Be specific. Here are a few examples of my daily affirmations.

"I have a positive attitude and think positive thoughts at all times."

"I am thorough, persistent and excellent in everything I do."

"I am physically healthy. I exercise for one hour every day, focusing on endurance, strength, and flexibility. I am confident and sexy!"

Do Not Disturb

I love this concept so much! I use "do not disturb" EVERY. SINGLE. DAY. I like to be able to focus on and be present in whatever I'm doing at the moment, and getting phone calls and texts a lot throughout the day is a huge distraction for me. It's extremely painful how distracting it is. Phone calls and texts are important and I have to respond, but I like responding on my own time when I'm ready. I am also a huge advocate for having airplane mode switch on at a certain time in the evening and then shut off at a certain time in the morning. So much stress comes from feeling like we don't have control of our own time, and that can happen when we let others dictate when and where we have conversations or talk about things. I know shutting your phone off seems little, but it can be a huge relief and keep the mind free from extra thoughts that don't need to be there.

GOAL: Set up automatic airplane mode for in the evening and early morning. Set up do not disturb for certain times throughout the day. This still allows you to receive texts and voicemails but doesn't notify you of them until you look at your phone which can correspond with your time blocks.

Brain Food

Taking supplements can be very beneficial in this day and age. The truth is that our food doesn't have quite as many nutrients as it did when the world first began. The processing of food and how long it takes to get it to our tables takes away important nutrients, so it's essential to not only fuel our bodies with good food but to understand that it may be necessary to fill in the gaps with supplements and vitamins. Taking vitamins like B12, vitamin D and magnesium especially can assist the health of the mind. Vitamins B12 and D are especially important for nerve health and fatigue. Magnesium is also beneficial to those who suffer from fatigue as well as those who run into anxiety problems.

GOAL: Talk to your doctor and see if you are deficient in any of these vitamins. Start taking them if you are. Try to get out of the mindset that you don't need vitamins or that you can get all of your nutrients from food. While that is the goal, and vitamins should NEVER replace good, hearty food, it also doesn't mean that you can't supplement your healthy food with some extra vitamins and minerals.

Visualization

We have all heard the saying "You win the morning, you win the day"; well, I'm here to say that it really does mean a lot to start strong and intentional in the morning, and when you do, it does carry over into the rest of your day. Self or day vision casting, or imagining your day before it actually happens, can be essential to how the day will play out. Although there are uncontrollable factors that can throw a kink in our plans, if we HAVE plans, we are at least trying to be intentional with the direction of our daily life. These tiny intentional moments carry over into the big picture, too.

I recently heard that Olympic gold medalists do this before a big event. They take a moment and envision themselves winning the medal before they actually do. They are intentional with their thoughts and take control of the outcome. You can do this, too. Envision the success of working out for forty-five minutes or nailing the big pitch meeting at work. Take control of your outcome before it happens!

GOAL: Before you step outside for the day or even move onto social media. Envision the success that you will have during your day—even in the little things—and then write them down. At the end of your day, go back to that list and see how much you accomplished by envisioning and focusing on it!

Example: I am articulate and will get verbal successful confirmation on the deal at work today. Envision your words and closing the deal at work before the meeting even happens or starts.

Be a Continual Learner

Life is constantly morphing around us, changing, expanding, and growing. Why do we resist change so much when it is inevitable? It's important to be a *learner*. This is someone who knows that they don't have it all figured out and, though they may be successful, still understands that they can learn from those around them. To be successful and to flourish in every area of our lives, we must learn from those who are already doing so. There are tons of experts in the world for a variety of skills, life hacks, and more. Go and learn from them. You can constantly better yourself in every area of life.

A great way that I do this is through podcasts or audiobooks which are convenient and allow me to learn while driving to work.

GOAL: Find a book from someone who is in a place that you want to be, physically, financially, emotionally, mentally, spiritually, relationally, etc. Start reading that book and applying those principles to your life. A great book to start with is The Slight Edge by Jeff Olson.

Get OUTSIDE

We spend a lot of our lives indoors with jobs, schooling and the increase of media in homes. There needs to be a balance and it's important to be outside just as much, if not more than we are inside. The sunshine, fresh air and break from media helps the body and mind to reset and restart. Getting outside in the sunshine allows your skin to absorb Vitamin D which is essential for bone strength and mental clarity and stability. Breathing the fresh air cleanses the nasal passages and refreshes the mind. Taking a break and stepping outside is essential to our sanity and well-being. It allows us to re-center our minds and can be used as a form of meditation.

Another way of meditation I use while being outside, is laying on my mat and watching the sky. It's relaxing to watch the clouds float by and the trees to sway in the breeze.

GOAL: Take a half hour each day from this day forward to be outside. Leave your phone or anything else that distracts you and just enjoy nature. Working in the garden, playing in the yard with kids, or walking the dogs are all great ways to get outside and clear the mind.

Stress

So many of us try to rid our lives of stress, which can honestly cause more stress. Instead of trying to get rid of stress completely, because that isn't realistic, try to cope with stress throughout your day and life. Realize that there will always be challenges in life and some are even beneficial to accomplishing growth. Stress can actually be helpful in some areas! Take, for example, working out. You put *stress* on your muscles when you work out but this encourages growth in the targeted muscle. The brain works the same way. So, channeling stress to benefit you instead of being fearful and paralyzed by it is going to help in the long run and increase your ability to handle stressful situations. Think of it as training your brain just like you trained your muscles in the last section. Implementing some breathing techniques or taking a moment away from the situation to think clearly, and then identifying the stress triggers so you know how to recognize them in the future and respond accordingly and successfully.

GOAL: Create a plan or list of a couple different coping mechanisms that you can implement the next time a stressful encounter comes your way. Be prepared to take action to stress instead of reacting and succumbing to it poorly. A great book to read in regard to this is "How to Stop Worrying and Start Living" by Dale Carnegie

Lifestyle

Relationships

The top stressor among people is home stress. This is unfortunate because your home is supposed to be the sanctuary you come to at the end of a long day. It's your peaceful haven, if you will. In order to maintain this peaceful haven, you need to care for the relationships in your home life. If you're married, your spousal relationship is your top priority and then children, and so on. Creating this environment comes from the direction and leadership that you hold in your home. It comes from creating boundaries as a family and deciding what your non-negotiables are. These will be the values that you hold in high regard in your home. These values should be implemented and carried out by each family member so as to maintain a healthy home. A couple examples of our family values are:

Standard of Honesty - *At all times and in all instances, we are truthful and honest towards each other even if it is difficult to say or hear. If one of us feels like there is an issue that is causing creeping separateness in the relationship they confront the other about it as soon as possible.*

Standard of Building Up - *We never put each other down in any way or in any circumstance even in joking. Instead, we constantly look for ways to build each other up publicly and privately.*

Remember, create these as a family so that it is easy to maintain them in to the future and so you are creating a sense of togetherness at the center of your values.

GOAL: Sit down with your spouse and family and write out your family values/non-negotiables as well as standards that you want to have for your home. If you are looking for more assistance on this, please email me at teliahgienger@gmail.com. I am more than happy to send you a copy of mine and Kylon's "Shield" if you need a template to get you and your family started!

Community

I'm sure you're familiar with the idea that you become the most like the five people you surround yourself with on a regular basis. This isn't to say that you become exactly like those people, but they influence you whether you realize it or not. It is important to surround yourself with people who motivate, encourage, challenge, and inspire you on a regular basis.

I don't think that this means you get rid of every friend who doesn't do those things for you, but I do think that this should stir some thoughts on who is in your life and whether they inspire growth or just bring gossip and negativity.

GOAL: Sit down and really evaluate the people in your life and how much time you're spending with them. Are they building you up and energizing you? Do they exhaust you and bring you down? These are important questions to ask. In order to create value in the world, you need to surround yourself with value. You are the average of the top five people you hang around.

Love What You Do

This is especially important after yesterday's entry. Just like surrounding yourself with people that build you up and encourage you, it's just as important to love what you do every day. If you don't love getting up every morning and putting in the work—maybe it's time to reevaluate. Reevaluating where the majority of my time is spent and if it's spent doing things I love and being with people that encourage growth in my life is something I love to do every year. If I'm not completely happy or in love with what I'm doing, I try to look for ways I can love it again or just find ways to eliminate what is making me NOT love it.

This may look like cutting back or hiring out some tasks that you normally do, or switching roles in the company. It's important that in this one life we live, we don't waste our time doing anything but completely loving every minute!

GOAL: Today's goal is to write down what takes up the majority of your time every day and evaluate if you truly love what you're doing and spending your time on. If not, write down the areas that you would like to change or shift around to excite you again.

You can break this up into "roles" if that's easier. For example: Wife, Husband, Mother, Father, Business Owner, Student, Sister, Brother, Friend, etc.

Create Connection

Connecting is the single greatest thing a human being can do. We are more capable than any other species to connect in the way we do. With that being said, connecting with someone means having a conversation. I mean real conversation about you and the person you are talking with. Getting to know someone is truly beautiful and something that doesn't happen as much as it should these days. A simple way of connecting with someone in conversation is by asking questions. Looking them straight in the eye and asking questions about them and their lives with sincerity. Connecting with someone is good for the heart and mind. It gets you out of your own space enough to realize that others have lives and are important. I find that it tends to put your "problems" into perspective and helps you to realize that they may not be that big of a deal.

GOAL: Today, your challenge is to connect with ONE person that you don't know. A complete stranger. Give them a smile and ask a simple question: "How are you doing today?" And then you listen. Continue talking with them naturally and wish them a good day. Along with that, I want to you notice their reaction when you talk to them with intention. I'll bet you just made their life better and that they'll remember that moment.

Give Back

As important as it is to get connected and learn from those around you, it's just as important to give back and teach. When you teach or share with someone else what you have learned or grown in, that skill or knowledge solidifies in your life even more. Find a group and give of yourself. The world thrives on learning and sharing, and it's your responsibility to do the same.

This encourages growth and inspires you to share the talents and knowledge that you have obtained over your life. Everyone has something to share and give, so what is yours?

GOAL: Today, write down all the areas that you feel you are well-versed in and have the ability to share with those around you. Then, write down how you can share those topics and through which platform. Online, in person, workshops, the possibilities are endless.

If you want to take this a step further, you can start today with a gift of your time to someone in need, a compliment, helping a stranger and even through the gift of money.

Be Intentional

Be intentional with the little decisions and know that they carry over into the rest of your life. This concept is one of my favorite practices and was developed after reading *The Slight Edge* by Jeff Olson. The idea is that every decision you make consistently compounds into the bigger picture of your life.

So, if you are making healthy decisions every day, you will most likely have long-term health habits. If you make tiny, consistent unhealthy choices, those will compound as well over time to create unhealthy habits.

GOAL: Write down five small choices that you can make today and every day hereafter that will compound into a healthy habit over time. Then, take those choices and post them somewhere you will see every day and often throughout the day as a reminder.

An example:

1. Drink 1 glass of water as soon as you wake up.

2. Step outside and breath 5 deep breaths in the morning.

3. Shut phone off at 7pm.

4. Walk/Jog for 10 minutes.

5. Be in bed by 10pm.

Have a Plan

Set goals and have a strategic plan for how you want your life to go. You have the ultimate control. I never use to be the type of person who wanted a plan, but as I grew up and my responsibilities grew, having a plan and setting goals became essential to seeing growth in my businesses and my personal life. My husband and I set family goals and relationship goals along with our business goals and every time we write one of them down, we accomplish them. It's because when you write a goal down, you're focusing on it and taking steps everyday to accomplish the larger objective.

GOAL: Sit down and write out your main goals for this year. Below each of those goals, what is your objective? Below the objective, what are the tasks that you need to complete to accomplish your objective and eventually your goal? Keep in mind, some goals can have more than one objective and more than one task for each objective. This will expand on your goal setting worksheet in the back of this book.

An example:

Objective: Lose weight.

Goal: Weigh ____ by September

Action Steps:

>   1. Run for 15 minutes 3 times a week

>   2. Track food and eat less than 1700 calories

>   3. Do bodyweight training 3 times a week

Minimalism

It's time to clean house. I'm not just talking literally either. I'm talking in every aspect of your life; you need to clear out the clutter. It's important to take time every couple of months and evaluate what is taking up space in your life that isn't providing value to you. I like to have a checklist of things that are taking up space and energy mentally, emotionally, spiritually, and physically in my life during these evaluation times.

If you can eliminate these things in your life every so often, you are keeping those important areas of your life clean and light. Free of clutter and free of distraction and free of potentially draining things.

GOAL: Sit down and make a list of each area of your life (you can separate by roles again.) and write down all of the things, people, and responsibilities you keep in those areas or roles. Then start going through and identify which ones are taking up space and which ones are motivating you.

Next step is simple: Eliminate everything that is just taking up space and energy. They are simply not necessary. Be ok with letting go of some things.

Break the Routine

This is such a great practice to have. Although I talk heavily on routine, especially when regarding our health, it's important to step outside our boxes and try new things. This may be a no-brainer for some, but some of us have to focus heavily on trying new things and stepping out. This practice, this focus on trying new things, can expand the brain and expand your knowledge of different cultures, viewpoints, and ultimately show you a new way of life. It doesn't even have to be anything huge, just get out there and try it! See how you feel, know what you don't like and what you love!

GOAL: Schedule something you have been looking to try but haven't yet. Just get out there and do it. Put it on the calendar, grab a friend and have fun!

Also, make sure that these new things are FUN and bring you joy!

Sleep

Growing up, I used to think that I didn't need sleep and that I shouldn't take naps because then I would be considered lazy. As I've gotten older and become more aware of what my body needs, I realize that naps are heavenly and that I do need a solid eight hours of sleep each night. My body will simply not function otherwise. Now, I don't think that every person needs eight hours. In fact, I think that each person has their own sleep needs and can function the way their body intended on different times of sleep. Take for instance my husband; he feels his best on 6.5-7 hours of sleep, whereas I need 8 as mentioned before. Recognizing what your body needs and accommodating isn't "lazy" or preventing you from accomplishing your day. In fact, I think it's the opposite. If you aren't getting enough sleep, you can't function properly and will most likely be tired and sluggish, or your brain might not be running at its peak because you're exhausted. Be aware though, that on the other side of this, too much sleep can make you feel even more tired. So, sleep well at night, and then get up and move. I have found that having a consistent bed time and wake up time is easy for me to maintain a healthy sleep pattern. Create a routine for yourself even with sleep and be consistent.

GOAL: Figure out how much sleep you need to function well throughout the day, set your routine bed times and wake up times and make sure you are getting good sleep! If you aren't, change it. Remember, YOU have the power over your life!

CONGRATULATIONS! You just finished the first 40 days of your new health journey!

Favorites and Resources

Recipes

Green Smoothie – Yields 16 oz

 ½ Cup Coconut Water

 1 Banana

 ½ Orange

 1 cup Kale

 1 cup Spinach

 ½ cup Frozen Blueberries

 5 Frozen Strawberries

 1 TBS Flaxseed OR Chia OR BOTH!

 Add: Ice if needed for thickness. If too thick, add more Coconut Water or regular water

Foundational Fruit Smoothie – Yields 16 oz

 ½ Cup Coconut Water/Tap Water

 1 Banana

 ½ Cup Raspberries

 ½ Cup Blueberries

 5 Frozen Strawberries

 Agave to sweeten

 Optional:

  1 Cup Spinach

1 TBS flaxseed OR chia OR BOTH!

Add: Ice if needed for thickness. If too thick, add more coconut water or regular water

Power Protein Smoothie – Yields 16 oz

½ Cup Almond Milk

1 Banana

2 TBS Almond Butter

1 TBS Agave

1 Scoop YOUR choice protein powder.

Here are a couple of my favorites:

MRM Protein Chocolate

Orgain Chocolate

Salad Dressing Recipe – Yields 2-2 ½ cups

1   package (16 ounces) frozen strawberries, thawed

6   tablespoons lemon juice

1/4 cup sugar

2   tablespoons cider vinegar

2   tablespoons olive oil

1/8 teaspoon poppy seeds

Directions: Place the strawberries in a blender; process until pureed. Add lemon juice and sugar; process until blended. While processing, gradually add vinegar and oil in a steady stream; process until thickened. Stir in poppy seeds. Transfer to a bowl or jar; cover and store in the refrigerator.

Favorite yoga routine

Seated Meditation: 8-10 min

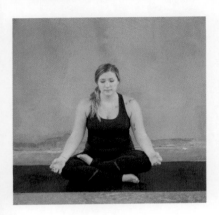

Seated Side Stretch -> Right Side/Left Side: Each side 8-10 breaths

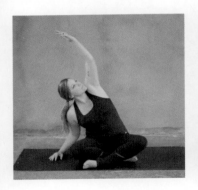 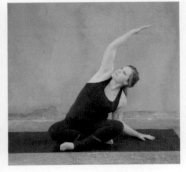

Seated Cat/Cow Breath

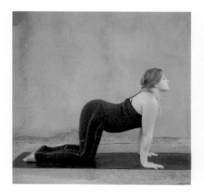 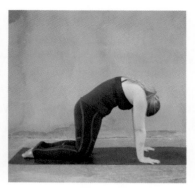

Boat Pose Crunches: 10 times

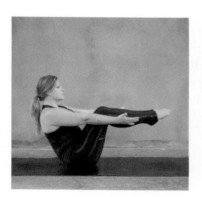 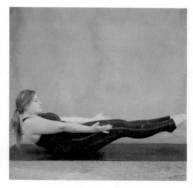

Downward-Facing Dog (Stretch/Walk out your heels feeling hamstring stretch)

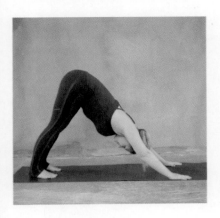

Surya Namaskar A (Sun Salutation A): 5 times

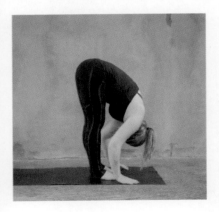

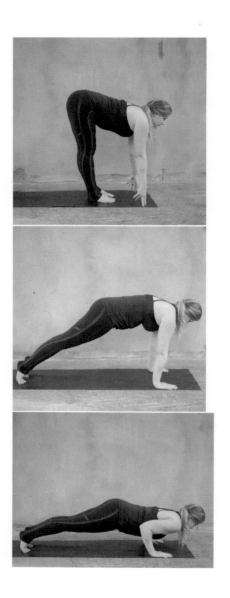

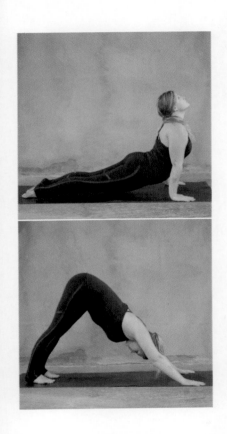

Walk to the top of mat dangle in rag doll

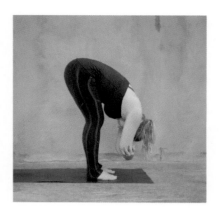

Extended Triangle -> Side Angle -> Half-Bind or Full Bind: Right Leg (REPEAT ON LEFT LEG)

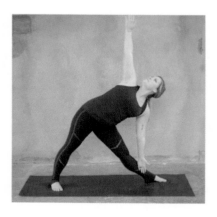

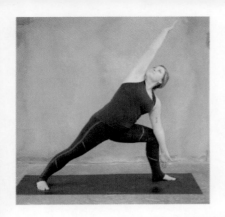

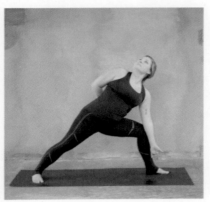

Wide-Legged Forward Fold -> Add in Shoulder rinse

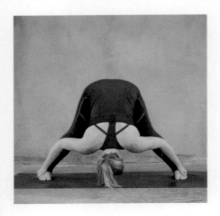

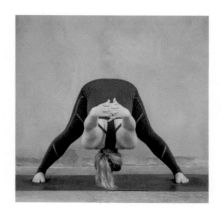

Sun Salutation A: 1 time

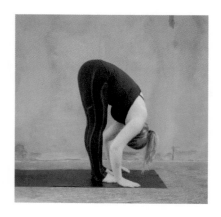

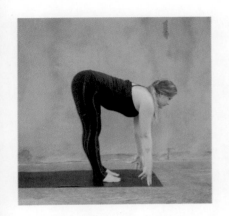

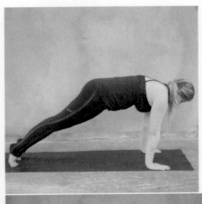

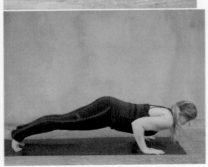

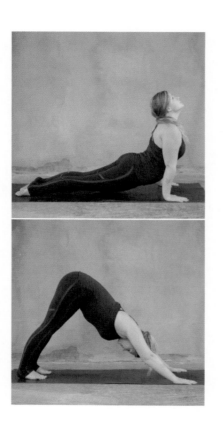

Dancing Warrior (1, 2, Reverse) – Right Leg/Left Leg: 2 times each side

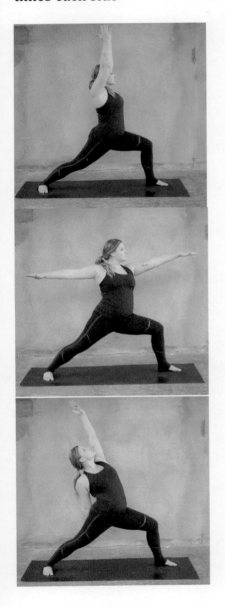

Bhujangasana (Cobra): 2 times

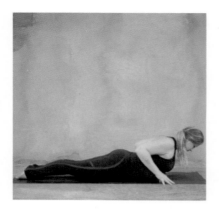

Salabhasana (Half-Locust): 2 times

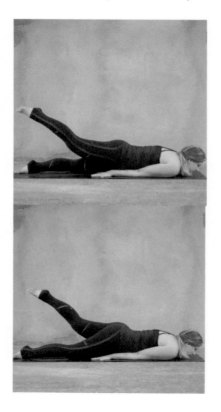

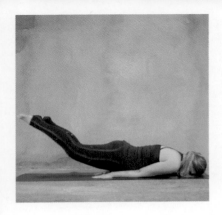

Poorna Salabhasana (Full Locust): 2 times

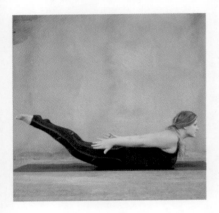

Dhanurasana (Floor Bow): 2 Times

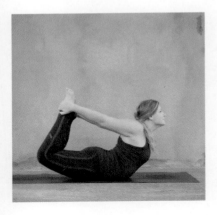

Ustrasana (Camel): 2 Times

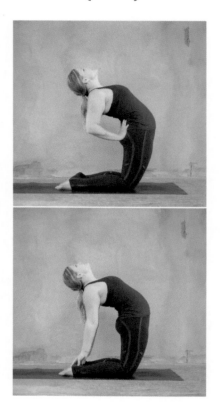

Bridge -> Full Wheel: 2 Times

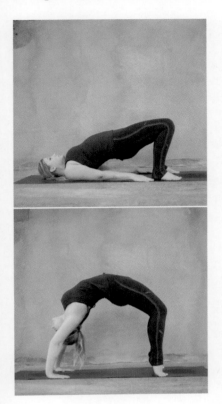

Lay on back -> Pull knees to chest

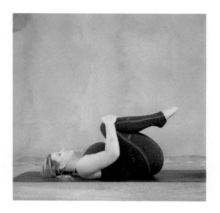

Happy Baby -> Savasana

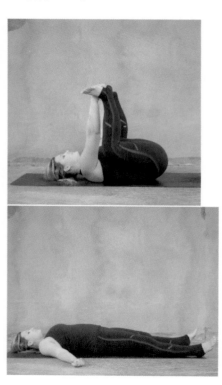

Favorite HIIT workouts

12 min AMRAP(As many rounds as possible)

Set a timer for 20 min (or less if you are in a hurry. Try to do at least 15 min)

> 30 Double Unders or 60 Single Jump Rope
>
> 10 Pushups
>
> 20 Crunches
>
> 15 Squats

Bodyweight workout – Repeat 3 times

> 30 Squats
>
> 20 Walking Lunges
>
> 10 Burpees
>
> 10 Inchworms
>
> 20 Curtsy Lunges
>
> 30 Pulsing Squats
>
> 10 Push-ups
>
> 20 Frog Crunches
>
> 30 Walking Lunges
>
> 10 Burpees
>
> 20 Bicycle Crunches
>
> 60 Second Plank

Tabata Workout - Start with 2 rounds of each circuit and build to 4 rounds

        Circuit 1

                Mountain Climbers – 20 Seconds

                10 Second Rest

                Push-ups – 20 Seconds

                10 Second Rest

        Circuit 2

                Side Lunges – 20 Seconds

                10 Second Rest

                Squats – 20 Seconds

                10 Second Rest

        Circuit 3

                High Knees – 20 Seconds

                10 Second Rest

                Jumping Jacks – 20 Seconds

                10 Second Rest

        Circuit 4

                Burpees – 20 Seconds

                10 Second Rest

                Flutter Kicks – 20 Seconds

                10 Second Rest

8 Minute Cardio Blast

        High Knees – 1 Min

        Squats – 1 Min

        Burpees – 1 Min

        Pushups – 1 Min

        Mountain Climbers – 1 Min

        Plank – 30 Seconds

        Lunges – 30 Seconds

Crunches – 30 Seconds

Side Crunches – 30 Seconds (15 seconds

each side)

Chair Dips – 1 Min

Favorite Meditation playlist

The Streets of Whiterun – Jeremy Soule

Walk – Ludovico Einaudi

Far Horizons – Jeremy Soule

Brothers – Ludovico Einaudi

Standing Stones – Jeremy Soule

Aurora – Jeremy Soule

Wind Guide You – Jeremy Soule

White Night – Ludovico Einaudi

Twenty Two Fourteen – The Album Leaf

Farewell to the Past – Ludovico Einaudi

The Light – The Album Leaf

The Earth - Ludovico Einaudi

Window – The Album Leaf

SMART Goal Worksheet

Today's Date: _____ Target Date: _____

Your Goal:

_____

Get SMART!

Specific: *What do you you want to accomplish (be painfully specific)*

_____

_____

Measurable: *How will you know when you have reached this goal?*

_____

_____

Achievable: *Is achieving this goal realistic with effort and commitment? Have you got the resources to achieve this goal? If not, how will you get them?*

_____

_____

Relevant: *Why is this goal significant to your life?*

_____

_____

Time Bound: *What is the date you will accomplish this goal?*

_____

This goal is important because:

_____

_____

The benefits of achieving this goal will be:

_____

_____

Take ACTION!

Specific Action Steps: *What steps need to be taken to get you to your goal?*

1:

2:

3:

4:

5:

Have Support!

Accountability Partners Names: *Who is cheering you on?* _____

_____

Thank you!

Thank you to everyone that helped me and inspired me in my health so I could one day write this book. To my mom, who always tried to "sneak" healthy items in our food so we wouldn't notice. You set the foundation of my living a healthy life. Also, we always noticed.

To my family, extended and immediate on every side that listens to me and asks my advice with yoga or health, you helped me find my voice and learn to communicate effectively.

To my businesses Renu and NUYU and my business partners Kennedy and Chelann, thanks for growing alongside me and inspiring me to be a better version of myself.

To my students and customers, thanks for giving me a way to look for new ways to be incorporate health in my life and the lives of our community.

To Kristi, the one that so meticulously edited this book for me when your schedule was so full of your own business. Thanks for being a true friend and a 'sister' after all of these years.

Finally, to my husband, Kylon. You are the biggest "thank you" of them all. Thanks for pushing me, inspiring me, working with me and helping me edit this book. You are such a big part of why I'm where I'm at today in business and life. I love you.

Printed in Great Britain
by Amazon

87276969R00045